CAREER AS A
PATHOLOGIST

MEDICAL DOCTOR

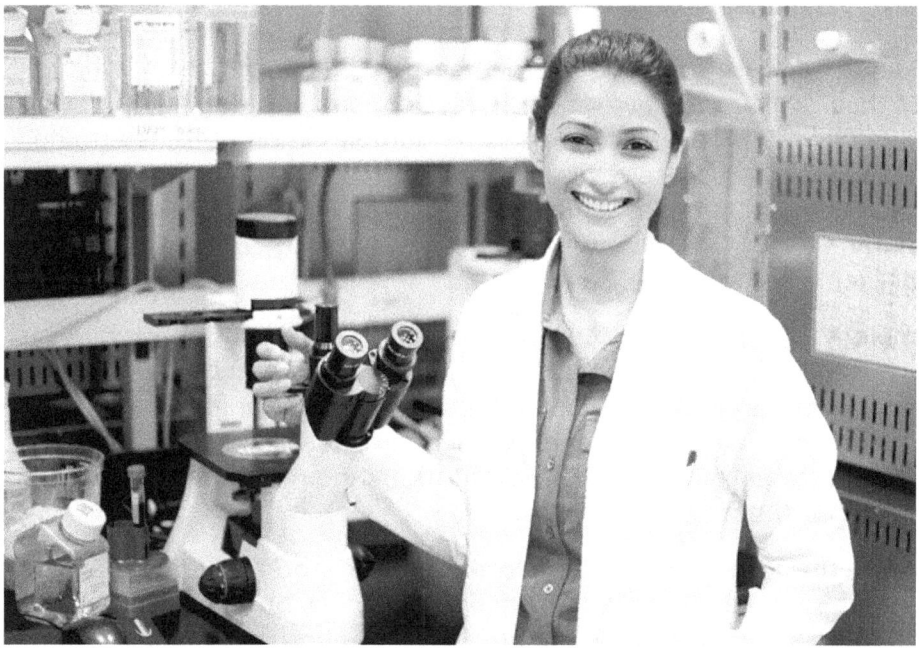

AN ELDERLY WOMAN IS FOUND unconscious in a supermarket aisle. Unresponsive, she is rushed to the emergency room. Upon regaining consciousness, she complains of a severe pain in her abdomen. There are many possible reasons for the pain, so a pathologist is called in to help solve the mystery. Blood and urine samples are taken and the pathologist examines them under a microscope. What the pathologist sees leads to a conclusive diagnosis. Now that the cause is known, the medical team can begin treatment.

Pathologists are like detectives, fascinated by the process of disease and dedicated to finding answers to medical mysteries. They use sophisticated tools and methods of modern laboratory science to identify and diagnose cancer, AIDS, diabetes, and many more diseases and health problems. Pathology literally means the study of disease, and consequently its scope is vast. Thousands of clinical, genetic, and microbiological tests are requested each day. It is the pathologist's job to examine tissue and body fluid samples, and provide expert interpretations of the results in order to facilitate diagnosis and treatment plans.

There are two main kinds of medical pathologists: clinical and anatomic. Clinical pathologists spend the majority of their time in the laboratory, examining blood, urine, and other body fluid samples in search of the cause of a disease. They are key members of the medical team, which uses their findings to diagnose and treat patients. Anatomic pathologists also analyze tissue and cell samples in order to determine the diagnosis and cause of diseases. The difference is the anatomic pathologist uses samples removed via surgery, biopsies, or fine needle aspirations. Their services are often needed urgently, while a patient is undergoing surgery.

Pathology is a very diverse field offering many different opportunities to practice in specific areas. There are many generalists, but most pathologists choose to focus on a specialty such as genetics, forensics, pediatrics, or molecular pathology. There are 10 such specialties in which a pathologist can obtain certification, and many more that can be practiced without certification.

Because the work is conducted primarily in the laboratory, it is ideal for individuals who are keenly interested in medicine, but have little desire for direct patient contact. Pathology labs are found in hospitals, colleges, and private companies that do medical research. Pathologists are employed by government agencies associated with agriculture, public health, law enforcement, and many other fields. Pharmaceutical companies and manufacturers of toxic substances like insecticides also employ pathologists.

The most successful pathologists are crack investigators and excellent communicators. They listen carefully as doctors describe symptoms and pay attention to every tiny detail while conducting lab tests. There is nothing routine about this work. Each case presents a new set of variables. The most valuable skill of all is the ability to recognize the common threads among diseases and visualize what is happening in a patient's body.

Are you ready to spend years studying and training, and a lifetime keeping up with advances in medicine? Becoming a pathologist entails one of the lengthiest education and training tracks of all physicians. The combination of undergraduate study, medical school, and residency add up to a dozen years or more. Certain subspecialties also require an additional year or two in a fellowship program.

In return for all the rigorous preparation, pathologists are rewarded with high salaries, excellent working conditions, and one of the only medical careers to feature normal 40-hour workweeks. If you are interested in the science behind medicine, want to work closely with other doctors, enjoy a balanced life, and solve the mysteries behind illness and deaths, pathology could be the career for you.

WHAT YOU CAN DO NOW

BECOMING A PATHOLOGIST TAKES many years of rigorous education. It is extremely important that you lay a good foundation early in high school. You should research college entrance requirements and ask your guidance counselor for help in putting together a curriculum that includes all the right courses. At the very least, you will need four years each of English, mathematics, and biological sciences. You should make every effort to make your high school years count by taking challenging courses in mathematics and the sciences. Look for AP courses, such as advanced placement chemistry, calculus, biology and physics.

Pathology demands good communication and writing skills. You can enhance those skills through classes in English composition, speech, drama, and debate. Psychology classes are useful for learning about human nature and exploring the mind-body connection. Classes in computer science are a plus.

Look for science clubs that involve laboratory work, research, and competitions. It is a great way to practice interacting with people of like interests, plus it will provide you the opportunity to become familiar with laboratory equipment and basic procedures.

During the summer months, many universities conduct summer study programs for high school students. These are generally month-long, tuition-free, residential programs, designed to improve academic study and communication skills. Some programs also offer internships that provide unique opportunities to interact with physicians and other healthcare professionals.

Volunteer opportunities exist year-round. The best places to volunteer are at health clinics, hospitals, women's clinics, or eldercare facilities.

Talk to medical pathologists in your community. You can find them by calling hospitals and universities. Your guidance counselor may be helpful in making connections, too. Talk to as many different kinds of pathologists as you can. Their advice is invaluable. Try to arrange to job shadow at least one pathologist to see what a working day in the field is really like.

Check out professional associations. Some, like the American Society for Clinical Pathology, offer information and resources for students interested in this career.

HISTORY OF THE PROFESSION

THE PRACTICE OF PATHOLOGY AS WE know it today is a complex application of advanced technology combined with a deep knowledge of human anatomy. Watching TV shows like House and CSI, it is hard to imagine that pathology existed before the computer. However, the rudimentary foundation for pathology was built long ago.

The story of pathology begins in ancient Egypt where papyrus documents contained information on different types of bone injuries, trachoma, ulcerating lumps, parasites, and other diseases. Several centuries later the study of disease was well underway in ancient Greece. Many notable physicians made lasting contributions to pathology, but none more than Hippocrates, who developed methods of diagnosis for a number of diseases. It was also in Greece that the practice of human cadaver dissection was first introduced. For many centuries, it was the dominant means for Greek physicians to learn anatomy. The practice slowly fell out of favor and ended with the burning of Alexandria in 389 AD. For more than 1,700 years, the European world valued the sanctity of the church more than scientific quests. It was not until the early 14th century that human dissection was revived as a tool for teaching anatomy in Bologna, Italy.

The influence of Hippocrates was evident in Roman medicine as well, and lasted until the Renaissance and beyond. Roman writers included in their texts remarkably clear descriptions of numerous pathological features, such as wound inflammation, tumors, hemorrhoids, malaria, and tuberculosis. The most important early Roman medical writer was Cornelius Celsus, who is best known for *De Re Medicina,* written in the first century. Contents of the encyclopedia covered numerous anatomy and pathology subjects, from the cause of disease to the diagnosis of internal maladies.

One of the greatest medical figures of all time was Roman physician Galen. Galen took the ideas of Hippocrates and developed Greco-Roman medical theory and practice. It is estimated that Galen wrote more than 500 books and treatises. His views on pathology were expressed in his books, *Seats of Diseases* and *Abnormal Tumors.*

Pathology emerged as a separate specialty during the Renaissance. It was a time of growth in the complex understanding of disease based on experimentation. The proliferation of scientific findings was largely unorganized and sporadically distributed until French physician Jean Fernel attempted to systemize the developing new knowledge in the 15th century. It was Fernel who introduced the term "physiology" to describe the study of the body's function. His main work, *Medicina*, contained a section called Pathologiae Libri, which became the standard medical text throughout Europe. In it, Fernal classified diseases as general and special ones, and distinguished symptoms and signs. His work was followed in the 16th century by several renowned anatomists who were increasingly aware of the pathological structures that they encountered during anatomical studies.

Many physicians in the 17th century studied diseases during autopsies, and some collected and published their findings. Of these early autopsy reports, the most important is Bonet's *Sepulchretum sive Anatomica Practica,* published in 1679. For this work, Swiss physician Theophile Bonet collected case descriptions of 3,000 autopsies performed over two centuries, including a few cases of his own. The two 1,700-page volumes were arranged in anatomical sections "from head to toe," with comments and references. The work is credited with opening the door to the modern practice of pathology. British physician Thomas Hodgkin offered a glimpse of the new pathology in 1836, when he wrote in his *Lectures on Pathologic Anatomy*: "Lister's compound microscope might lead to useful discoveries in the future."

Modern Pathology

Medicine advanced in the 18th century. Many pathologic observations were published in textbooks and journals. Yet, modern pathology was not established as a distinct field of science until the 19th century and did not fully develop until the early 20th century, with the advent of detailed study of microbiology. In the 19th century, physicians began to understand that disease-causing pathogens, or "germs" existed. With the new understanding of causative agents, physicians began to compare the characteristics of different germs and their related symptoms in affected individuals.

The biggest single advancement in the development of pathology was the compound microscope, which could be used to analyze tissues. The new device completely refocused the study of disease from whole organs to cells, which marked the beginning of a new pathology. With the emergence of microscopy, medical schools throughout Europe began to add professors of pathology to their faculties for the first time.

From the mid-19th century onwards, rather than the work of any one individual, it was new technology that shaped the field of pathology. Starting at the beginning of the 20th century, the pace of research in pathology greatly accelerated. The number of discoveries since has grown exponentially, along with the number of scientists and doctors devoted to the field of study.

By the early 1930s, pathology was deemed a medical specialty. The field began to split into a number of esoteric fields, resulting in the development of a large number of subspecialties within pathology. Ongoing advances have continued to yield better diagnostic tools, and better, more precise diagnoses. Many new journals appeared to report new findings and techniques, including subspecialty journals covering the broadest array of pathology.

Over a span of 4,000 years, concepts of medicine and disease have changed. In the never-ending search for the cause of disease, the earliest physicians looked at the human body as a whole, and often referred to the will of the gods, the stars, and other invisible forces. More recently, medical knowledge in general, and pathology in particular, have been driven by the relentless progress of technology.

Today, powerful new technologies are forcing yet another revision of pathology ideas, from cell-based disease, to gene-based disease, to individual molecules and their interplay. Pathology is a vital part of the medical field that will continue to grow in coming years due to the emergence of new diseases every year. In the future, to combat these new diseases there will be improvements in disease detection, treatment, and classification. A big factor will be genome-based laboratory testing and disease research, which promises to provide more precise and accurate detections of disease.

WHERE YOU WILL WORK

THERE ARE APPROXIMATELY 15,000 board certified pathologists working in the United States today. It is a broad field with a variety of different types of employers. Hospitals, medical schools, the military, and government agencies employ most medical pathologists. With the growth of ambulatory care, an increasing number of pathologists practice in non-hospital settings, such as private or group practices, clinics, and other healthcare facilities.

Pathologists most often work in hospitals where they are considered the "doctor's doctor" because of their vital input for making diagnosis, treatment, and health management decisions. About 75 percent of pathologists practice in the community hospital setting, though many other options exist. In a community hospital practice, the pathologist contributes to medical decisions related to all medical specialties on the hospital staff. Hospital pathologists often operate laboratories that also serve the office practices of physicians in the community. As laboratory director, the pathologist is involved in quality improvement, risk management, continuing medical education, and development of comprehensive information systems.

Another large employer of pathologists are medical schools. There are about 3,000 pathologists working on college and university campuses, where they lecture in classrooms and conduct basic or applied research. A small number serve as deans and as members of national professional and research bodies.

Many pathologists work in the military and in government agencies. These government agencies are usually related to public health, agriculture, and law enforcement, among others. The National Institutes of Health, Armed Forces Institute of Pathology, and Food and Drug Administration are among the largest employers of pathologists of all kinds. Forensic pathologists are employed by municipal, state, and federal agencies, where they investigate unexplained and unnatural deaths.

A growing number of independent laboratories are hiring pathologists. Many of these labs are part of large national medical networks. Others are regional or local. In addition, pathologists are found in research institutes and working with pharmaceutical and biotechnology companies. Some private companies, such as those who manufacture drugs and insecticides, also employ pathologists.

Pathology is a broad field. Conditions vary depending on the working environment. Most pathologists spend some time in laboratories. Like most scientific or medical research facilities, pathology labs are typically well equipped with the latest technology, such as electron microscopy and computer modeling. Many pathologists work at least part of the time in offices or in classrooms. Depending on their field, pathologists may also spend time in greenhouses, on farms, in hospital wards, or in morgues.

For most pathologists, the basic 40-hour workweek is the norm. How those hours are scheduled, however, will vary according to the type of employer. For example, those working in hospitals may work rotating shifts. Shift work usually amounts to the same 40 hours even though the scheduling is flexible. In general, the hours for pathologists are usually shorter and more regular than those of physicians who have their own practices.

THE WORK YOU WILL DO

PATHOLOGY IS A MEDICAL SPECIALTY that provides the scientific foundation for all medical practice. Although the areas of practice are very different, pathologists are all scientists who study disease. Since all pathologists are also doctors, pathology is known as the bridge between basic science and medicine.

Pathology is the study of blood, fluid, and tissue samples in order to determine the cause of illness or death. The pathologist's findings are most often used to make diagnoses by looking for specific factors lacking or present in the samples. In medical care, the pathologist is a very valuable part of the medical team, since many diseases are diagnosed or ruled out by microscopic and lab analysis of fluid or tissue samples. The pathologist works with all other medical specialties, using the tools of laboratory medicine, such as cytology and histology to provide essential information.

Pathology is generally divided into two main areas: clinical and anatomic. Clinical pathology is the study of disease and disease processes. The work is conducted primarily in the laboratory, where clinical pathologists analyze bodily fluids such as blood and spinal fluid, as well as bodily tissues and even individual cells. The lab results are used to support the diagnosis of disease for patients needing treatment. For example, a pathologist might use the tools of microbiology to identify a microorganism that could be causing an infection in a sick patient. Many of these microorganisms – bacteria, fungi, viruses, and parasites – can only be seen using a powerful microscope. Once the microorganism is identified, the clinical pathologist cannot only declare a diagnosis, but also make recommendations for the most appropriate treatment.

Anatomic pathology is the study of the structural and functional changes in cells, tissues, and organs that underlie disease. Most often, the anatomic pathologist is examining surgical specimens removed from the body during operations. Surgeons often need immediate diagnoses on biopsies. There is often an anatomic pathologist (also known as a surgical pathologist) standing by to receive tissue samples or cellular fluids while the patient remains under anesthesia. The pathologist must quickly, but thoroughly, process the samples and provide information vital to the successful conclusion of a surgery in progress. Anatomic pathology also involves the examination of the whole body during autopsy. The same tools and procedures are used to investigate and determine the cause of death.

Work Duties

The pathologist's role in medical practice is central to patient care, although they usually do not treat patients of their own. Their work is more behind the scenes and they rarely, if ever, meet a patient. As consulting physicians, they provide essential information to clinical colleagues, such as surgeons, radiologists, and primary care physicians. Their vital input is used to make diagnosis and treatment decisions, and form the foundation for future health management.

Pathologists may prepare specimens themselves, but the routine laboratory tests are often conducted by a team of medical laboratory technologists or technicians. In that case, the pathologists oversee the functioning of the laboratory and supervise the team. They are also responsible for quality control and safety, particularly in the processing and storage of blood samples and products in the lab or in blood banks.

Pathologists also do scientific research into drugs and diseases. Pharmaceutical companies developing new drugs need pathologists to study their efficacy and safety. Pathologists use microscopes, radioisotopes, and other scientific methods and computerized data to analyze and test theories about the processes of diseases and the possible therapeutic effects (and side effects) of drug therapies.

Teaching is often part of the pathologist's job. They impart their knowledge to their medical colleagues through consultations and formal seminars. They sometimes conduct in-house seminars for hospital staff and interns. Those who are college and medical school faculty members teach classes attended by students of nursing, medicine, laboratory technology, and other healthcare subjects. They also teach law enforcement officers how to use scientific methods to investigate injuries or deaths.

Specialization

Because of its broadly diverse nature, pathologists are able to select a niche that best suits their needs. Many pathologists are generalists who deal with all facets of disease. Others have particular interests and specialize in narrowly focused areas. For the latter, there are 10 certification subspecialties in pathology to choose from. Some master all or at least several subspecialties for more diverse work and a more flexible career path. Some are subspecialists in anatomical pathology, others are clinical.

Transfusion Pathology

Blood banking and transfusion involves the maintenance of an adequate blood supply, blood donor and patient-recipient safety, and appropriate blood utilization. The blood donor center is the facility that collects and processes blood products. The pathologist oversees the collection and subsequent processing and distribution by the blood bank. Transfusion medicine (transfusiology) is also concerned with blood donation, but encompasses issues of immunohematology, therapeutic apheresis (the removal of harmful proteins, chemicals, or cells in the blood that contribute to disease), stem cell collections, cellular therapy, and coagulation. Pathologists who specialize in transfusion medicine are expert in transfusion practices, and are often responsible for pretrans-fusion compatibility and antibody testing to assure that blood transfusions are as safe as possible.

Chemical Pathology

Chemical pathology is concerned with the biochemical basis of disease and the use of biochemical tests for screening, diagnosis, prognosis and management. Pathologists in this area typically test for concentrations of electrolytes, metabolites, proteins, and hormones. They also measure markers of liver and kidney function, and tumors. Test results are used in the management of a wide range of conditions and metabolic disorders such as cancer, diabetes, high cholesterol, liver disease, and kidney stones. Chemical pathologists are also expert in toxicology, therapeutic drug monitoring, and detection of illicit drugs and poisons.

Cytopathology

Cytopathology involves the study and diagnosis of disease on the cellular level. The first and most widely known cytopathology test is the Pap test, which is used to screen for cervical cancer. Cytopathology techniques are applied to all organ systems and their diseases. A cytopathologist looks for disease in individual cells. The cell samples may be in smears, aspirates, or body fluids.

A specialized form of cytopathology is fine needle aspiration biopsy, a diagnostic procedure used to investigate lumps or masses. It involves inserting a thin needle into an area of abnormal-appearing tissue or body fluid. The sample collected can help make a diagnosis or rule out conditions such as cancer.

Dermatopathology

Dermatopathology is concerned with diseases of the skin. Dermatologists are usually able to identify cutaneous diseases based on appearance, anatomic distribution, and behavior. However, some cases require information that the human eye cannot see. The dermapathologist can make a more conclusive diagnosis by examining samples from a skin biopsy. In addition to microscopic examination, specialized testing at the molecular level may be needed to provide a specific diagnostic interpretation.

Forensic Pathology

Forensic pathology is focused on determining the cause of death by examining a corpse. The practice can be anatomic or clinical. Sometimes postmortem examinations (autopsies) are performed because the cause of death is unclear. The information may be needed by criminal investigators to determine possible criminal involvement in a person's death.

An anatomic forensic pathologist may serve as a consultant to the coroner or be the appointed medical examiner. Clinical forensic pathologists examine both living and deceased individuals. They can evaluate the extent to which treatment had helped a patient, giving valuable information to physicians caring for other patients with similar conditions.

Hematology

Hematology is the study of blood, the blood-forming organs, and blood diseases. By analyzing abnormal blood smears, hematologists can identify problems such as clotting and other bleeding disorders, leukaemias, and anaemias. As experts, they may also be asked to supervise the treatments. In some cases, they collect bone marrow specimens from patients. They may also be responsible for blood banking and for interpreting and advising others on the meaning of various blood tests.

Medical Microbiology

Medical microbiology is concerned with the prevention, diagnosis, and treatment of infectious diseases. Medical microbiologists look for bacteria, viruses, and parasites. They may examine tissues or fluid from any part of the human body. Their primary goal is to identify and stop the spread of contagious disease. For example, they may be responsible for controlling the spread of hospital-acquired infections, such as Staphylococcus aureus or norovirus. In the hospital setting, these specialists also help in the management of wound infection after surgeries, as well as infections associated with catheters and IVs.

Molecular Pathology

Molecular pathology is the study and diagnosis of disease through the examination of molecules within organs, tissues, or bodily fluids. The molecules studied are DNA, RNA, and protein. Molecular pathology is commonly used in the diagnosis of solid tumors (cancer), hereditary diseases such as cystic fibrosis, hematologic malignancies (leukemia), and infectious diseases such as HIV/AIDS.

Neuropathology

Neuropathology is concerned with diseases of the nervous system, both central (brain and spinal cord) and peripheral (nerves). By examining samples obtained from small surgical biopsies or whole body autopsies, neuropathologists are able to detect tumors in the brain and spinal cord, viruses and bacteria, and neurodegenerative disorders like

Alzheimer's disease and Huntington's disease. They can also determine how the nervous system is reacting to traumatic causes.

Pediatric Pathology

Pediatric pathology is devoted to the laboratory diagnosis of diseases that occur in children.

A pediatric pathologist looks for diseases and disorders that could impact the normal growth and development of children from the embryonic stage to adolescence.

Pathologists With no Medical Degree

Though most pathologists have medical degrees, there are a few exceptions. People with a degree in dental medicine may examine collected body samples from the mouth to diagnose dental illness. Veterinarians and zoologists can also specialize in pathology and diagnose the illness of animals. Plant pathologists (sometimes called phytopathologists) are botanists who diagnose and manage plant diseases.

STORIES OF WORKING PATHOLOGISTS

I Am a Forensic Pathologist

"I have carried out more than 2,000 autopsies during my professional career. It is my job to determine the cause and manner of death in situations falling under the jurisdiction of the coroner or medical examiner. Some of these deaths are violent, such as car crashes, suicides, and homicides. Most aren't necessarily violent, but are suspicious because they are sudden and unexpected. They include deaths in infants and children, deaths that occur after surgeries, and situations where illicit drug use is suspected. These are just a few examples. One of the most important and interesting reasons for an autopsy is when there is suspicion of a public health threat. Studying the dead is the only way to determine the most effective clinical management of a disease. Many diseases unknown for centuries were only discovered through postmortem examination.

In addition to performing autopsies, I spend time acquiring data from witnesses and investigating officers, testifying in court, and writing reports. Occasionally I visit scenes of accidents or crimes, but despite what you see on TV, that is uncommon. My days are long. Unlike most other pathologists, my hours are not limited. For me, 10 to 12 hours or longer are not unusual.

Becoming a forensic pathologist was not easy. My education and training after graduating from high school took 13 years. Obviously, only someone who has an intense interest in the field would want to make that investment. I was hooked the moment I sat down in a pathology elective class and peered into a microscope. Over the years, I have experienced a great deal of professional satisfaction. The work is challenging and exciting, and I feel that I am making an important contribution to the community.

My advice to anyone considering pathology is to keep in mind that you will be a physician first and foremost. Include in your medical school elective blocs an autopsy pathology rotation as early as possible. You will know right away if forensics appeals to you and if it does, you will have a head start on the first day of residency. You should also choose your residency carefully. I strongly suggest a program associated with a university, not a private hospital."

I Am a Consultant Hematologist

"As a consultant I have several roles. I teach undergraduate classes, work part time for a transfusion service, and spend two days a week at a local care center for hemophilia. I also manage the care for patients taking long-term warfarin (an anticoagulant used to prevent heart attacks, strokes, and blood clots). Unlike most pathologists, my work includes a high level of patient contact. That is my choice – a choice I can make because I am a consultant.

My interest in pathology came during my second year of medical school. My father was a surgeon and I always knew I wanted to go into medicine, but it wasn't until I realized I was really enjoying my neuroscience class that I considered moving away from clinical practice. Pathology is very much the scientific end of medicine. And hematology is relevant across medicine, surgery, and the many specialties. For me, it's been the perfect choice.

It was during my residency that I became interested in being a consultant. In medicine, a consultant is an expert who is called in to give a fresh perspective and provide a diagnosis or opinion. The importance of the consultant pathologist's diagnosis can't be understated. Very often, the entire medical team and their course of treatment are solely dependent on information provided by the pathologist. This faith in the pathologist is not misplaced. Pathologists have a profound knowledge of virtually every disease process that can affect every organ. It's no wonder that the opinions of consulting pathologists are so highly regarded.

Pathology is intellectually challenging. It is a subject that encompasses all medical sciences, including anatomy, histology, physiology, genetics, biochemistry, epidemiology, and clinical medicine. The challenge makes medicine both exciting and alive for me. It is complex and ever changing. I am constantly studying and learning more. Boredom is simply not possible.

Aspiring pathologists should work hard in high school, develop good study habits, and practice self-discipline. Do that, and college and med school will go more smoothly. Early on, look into joining at least one pathology association. Attending their conferences is the best way to gain access to med school faculty members and pathologists of different specialties. The knowledge you can gain from them is invaluable."

PERSONAL QUALIFICATIONS

PATHOLOGISTS ARE FUNDAMENTALLY medical doctors. The main difference between most pathologists and physicians is pathologists are far less likely to be involved in direct patient care. Are you drawn to the scientific, analytical, and technical aspects of medicine? If so, pathology may be what you are looking for. It is an ideal career for someone who is intensely interested in medicine, but prefers to work in a lab behind a microscope rather than meeting with patients all day.

Pathologists must have an aptitude for science. Their interest cannot be limited to biology, anatomy, and physiology. Physics, chemistry, and the social sciences, such as anthropology and psychology, are also important to the work.

A good eye for spatial relationships is necessary to become a good pathologist. Pathology is a visual specialty and some people are more suited to it than others. What pathologists see using a microscope are not just colored structures, but patterns. Starting with innate visual ability, they are trained to utilize that talent to recognize more and more patterns. It takes time and experience, but eventually they get to the point where they can build pictures in their minds. Mastering this talent is one of the reasons why the training takes so long.

Good communications skills, both speaking and writing, are essential. Pathologists of all kinds spend time planning projects, attending meetings, and discussing findings with physicians and other scientists. Those specializing in forensics often have to interact with law enforcement officers, first responders, and civilian witnesses. Confidence and a knack for persuasion can come in handy for these specialists on the occasions they must convince judges and juries that their findings are valid.

Pathology is intellectually challenging. It requires observational skills and a methodical approach to work. Attention to detail is critically important. Pathologists are necessarily careful and precise, especially when a diagnosis is crucial for determining the direction of patient care. A pathologist's opinion may affect whether a relatively simple or noninvasive treatment will be sufficient, or if someone will need a radical procedure or toxic chemotherapy. Good pathologists are also thorough in their thinking. They have the ability to absorb a great deal of information and the patience to complete lengthy research projects.

Do you enjoy solving mysteries? A good pathologist has the mind of a detective. Discovering rare and sometimes unknown causes of illness or death is what successful pathologists thrive on.

This work requires a strong stomach. For many pathologists, autopsies are part of the daily routine. Those in forensic pathology have it the worst. They have to deal with dismembered and sometimes rotting bodies.

ATTRACTIVE FEATURES

PATHOLOGISTS ARE PAID VERY WELL. Starting salaries are well into the six-figure range and the overall average is more than $250,000 a year. Some subspecialties, especially when practiced in a major university hospital, yield up to $100,000 more than the average. Pathologists who work in a private practice or have consulting practices can also earn well above the average. Yet as good as that sounds, career satisfaction is not usually about the money. In fact, only 10 percent of pathologists say that the most rewarding aspect is making good money. About three out of four pathologists say that being good at what they do and providing critical information that is used in healing and saving lives of patients are the most satisfying aspects of their work.

Pathologists enjoy a myriad of opportunities. Within the field, there is a very wide and endless variety in the work for both generalists and specialists. Generalists can have a broad focus across all human organs and systems, instead of just one, like most clinicians. They can also narrow their focus and choose to work in any one area of medicine. There are numerous specialties and subspecialties. Currently, there are 10 different certifications available, plus more subspecialties that are practiced without additional certification.

The medical field is notorious for consuming most, if not all, of a physician's time. The story is very different for most pathologists. A 40-hour workweek is the norm, which allows for a balanced and fulfilling life. Only occasionally are pathologists on call and they are rarely called in at night. (The only exception is for forensic specialists.) While the demands are not nearly as pressing as those in other disciplines, there is the potential to have a life-saving impact on patients.

The work is very challenging, but it is also very interesting. Pathologists report that 90 percent of their work is interesting and only 10 percent is tedious. That is the opposite of what most physicians experience. Few medical specialties offer seeing something new every day, but pathology is a process of continual discovery.

The pathologist is an essential member of the clinical team. How the patient will be treated and what the outcome will be often depends on the pathologist's diagnosis. The pathologist usually doesn't treat patients directly, but rather interacts with other members of the clinical team. These continuous interactions are intellectually very stimulating.

UNATTRACTIVE ASPECTS

A LENGTHY AND RIGOROUS EDUCATION is required. After high school come four years of college, then four years of medical school, followed by four or five years of residency. The training continues for those pursuing certain subspecialties. They need to spend an additional year or two in a fellowship program. That is a minimum of 12 years and possibly as many as 15 years spent preparing for a career in pathology. Of course, beginning with the residency, you will be employed and earning a salary.

The loss of direct patient contact is a drawback for some pathologists. Much of the work is done out of sight, where your efforts are usually unknown to patients and their families. Only the doctors who consult the pathologists know how vital their work is. Prestige is afforded to more visible practitioners, such as surgeons. Because there are so many different ways to practice pathology, the option to work directly with patients does exist for some who want to, although this is not the norm.

EDUCATION AND TRAINING

THE EDUCATION REQUIRED TO BECOME a pathologist is long and rigorous. Pathologists hold at least two degrees, a bachelor's degree and a medical degree. It takes about eight years to get that far. In some cases they spend six years in medical school in order to earn a doctoral degree in pathology in addition to their medical degree.

The training requirements do not stop there. It also takes at least four to five years of post-graduate training in a pathology residency to qualify to sit for the board certification exam. For certain subspecialties, another one or two years in a fellowship program follows. Medical pathologists are likely to spend a total of at least 12 years in training before they are fully qualified in their profession.

Undergraduate Study in Pathology

Following high school, the first step to become a pathologist is to earn a bachelor's degree from a four-year college or university. The goal is to prepare for admission to medical school. Any undergraduate major is acceptable, but the most advantageous are biology, chemistry, or a related science field. Those who choose other majors should at least take courses in biology, chemistry (including general chemistry, organic chemistry, and biochemistry), physics, mathematics, and English. It is important to pay particular attention to the required courses for medical school admission. The list of required science courses, for example, is quite specific at most medical schools.

There are a number of qualities that medical schools look for in applicants. First is academic achievement in college. In addition to a high grade point average, a good score on the Medical College Admissions Test (MCAT) is expected. The MCAT is required for admission to any medical school. Admissions officers will also look for extracurricular activities, leadership, community service, research, and patient exposure. The last item can be obtained by volunteering at hospitals, participating in internships, or shadowing multiple physicians.

To find a medical school, consult the Liaison Committee on Medical Education (LCME). A list of 135 accredited medical programs in the US is listed on the organization's website.

Graduate Studies

Medical school is a four-year training program that consists of two parts: two years of basic science instruction and two years of clinical instruction. The basic science instruction, which is covered in the first two years, includes courses in anatomy, physiology, biochemistry, histology, immunology, microbiology, and pathology. Classes also cover anatomy and bodily systems, and major diseases.

Students get practical hands-on experience outside the classroom during the third and fourth years. Instruction is generally provided through clinical rotations in various areas of medicine. The purpose of medical school is to provide a foundation for all kinds of physicians, not just pathologists. In most cases, pathology is not a required rotation and must be taken as an elective.

Residency Training

The next step in becoming a pathologist is to undergo further training as a medical resident. A residency is advanced medical training in a specialized field. Residents work under the supervision of a licensed medical doctor. Pathology residencies last four to five years, and are among the longer residencies a doctor may choose. By contrast, an internal medicine residency lasts three years. Pathology residents are compensated for their time with modest salaries and other benefits, such as health insurance.

Most pathology residents train in both anatomic pathology (AP) and clinical pathology (CP), although it is possible to train in only one. During training, the resident becomes familiar with all activities of a pathology department, with instruction in autopsy, cytogenetics, image analysis, molecular diagnostics, and protein biochemistry. Residents are also given opportunities to participate in research projects.

Fellowships

Pathologists who plan to practice in subspecialty areas such as dermatopathology, surgical pathology, or pediatric pathology need to complete a fellowship. Fellowship programs usually last a year or two. The training is more narrowly focused than that received during residencies. Some fellowships may include additional rotations in different areas. For example, a surgical pathology fellowship may include rotations in gastrointestinal, breast, soft tissue, and gynecologic pathology.

Fellows are licensed medical doctors who are working usually in close tandem with one or more experienced pathologists, as they enhance their knowledge and hone their abilities in a particular area.

Licensure and Certifications

To practice pathology, those who have completed their residencies must become licensed by passing the United States Medical Licensing Examination to become a medical doctor, or the Comprehensive Osteopathic Medical Licensing Exam to become an osteopathic doctor. A license will also be required by the state in which you plan to practice.

Pathologists also need to be board certified. This entails passing written and practical exams offered by the American Board of Pathology (ABP).

The ABP publishes a booklet of information on board certification and requirements. Generally, certifications may be in combined clinical and anatomic pathology, anatomic pathology, or clinical pathology.

There are also options for certification in 10 different subspecialties:

- Blood banking and transfusion
- Chemical pathology
- Cytopathology
- Dermatopathology
- Forensic pathology
- Hematology
- Medical microbiology
- Molecular genetic pathology
- Neuropathology
- Pediatric pathology

Continuing Education

Pathologists need to meet continuing medical education requirements and professional performance standards in order to maintain certification.

EARNINGS

THE MEDSCAPE PHYSICIAN COMPENSATION REPORT reports average annual compensation for pathologists at $267,000. This represents a 12 percent increase over the average pathologist's compensation of $239,000 just one year previously. As part of their annual compensation, pathologists also earn an average of $10,000 for non-patient related activities. That makes pathologists among the highest salaried professionals in the field of medicine.

Overall, average salaries for certified pathologists cover a wide range, from a low of about $150,000 to more than $350,000 based on experience, geographic location, and the kind of job. The lower end of the scale generally reflects starting salaries for newly certified pathologists. The highest salaries are paid to well-established professionals.

Pathologists working in hospital laboratories earn a higher annual income compared to those working in private companies or practices.

Some of the best paying cities for pathologists in the United States include Seattle, Houston, New York,   and Los Angeles. Statewide, pathologists in Minnesota enjoy the highest pay levels. Regionally, pathologists earn the most in the North Central and Southeast. The lowest earners live in the Northeast and the Mid-Atlantic regions. Even in those locations, the average salaries are generally above $250,000 annually.

The biggest differences in compensation for pathologists are found among the various work settings. The highest paid pathologists out-earn the lowest paid by over $150,000 annually. Here is how the average annual earnings compare:

- Office-based, multi-specialty, group practices
  $356,000

- Office-based, single-specialty, group practices
  $327,000

- Healthcare organizations
  $270,000

- Hospitals
  $265,000

- Office-based solo practices
  $260,000

- Academic (non-hospital), military, research, and government employers
  $185,000

Some pathologists choose to practice as independent consultants. These self-employed individuals earn significantly more than their salaried colleagues do. The income differential is significant, estimated to be over 35 percent. That is more than enough to compensate for the additional expenses such as self-employment tax and health insurance that must be self-funded. Salaried pathologists usually receive benefits that include paid holidays and vacations, health insurance, and retirement plans. Self-employed pathologists do not receive benefits.

OPPORTUNITIES

THE JOB OUTLOOK FOR PATHOLOGISTS is very good. The only factor that may limit demand is advances in technology. If there is any impact at all, it is likely to be small. Pathology is very much a hands-on practice that requires the kind of complex judgments only a highly trained professional can make.

Jobs will be plentiful in large hospitals, medical centers, and private practices located in urban areas. However, that is also where job seekers will find the most competition. The best opportunities will be in rural, low-income, or underserved communities, which have a hard time attracting doctors of any kind.

Pathologists are generally eager to work in academia, not necessarily because they want to teach, but more because they want to get involved in important university-sponsored research projects. However, the interest in that area has created growing competition for jobs in universities. Most new research jobs for pathologists will be offered by private research firms and medical laboratories. Private industry, in general, is a growing source of new jobs. As a result of increased interest in preserving the environment, expanding food supplies, and improving healthcare, private companies are expected to devote funds to research in pathology.

The primary reason for the increasing demand for pathologists is the need to serve a growing elderly population. The elderly are particularly susceptible to diseases like cancer. Medical pathologists, who are instrumental in diagnosing cancer, will be required in greater numbers as a result.

Job growth will vary by subspecialty. The public has been intrigued with forensics for years, mostly because of popular TV shows like CSI that appeal to the innate human fascination with the macabre and the love of a good detective story. That does not mean forensics is the best choice for new pathologists. The fact is, forensics represents only a very small number of jobs, and the subspecialty currently has more doctors than are required. On the other hand, there are not enough medical students preparing for a career in pathology to keep up with demand in other areas. There is a shortage of pathologists, particularly in sub-specialties such as hematology, microbiology, and immunology. Pathology students should carefully consider which subspecialty to pursue, taking into consideration future career opportunities.

A relatively new career path in clinical pathology is medical informatics. This is where skills in both medical and computer sciences work together. Over the past few decades, there has been a great expansion in medical information in general. This is partly due to legal requirements, but also because of the complex interactions involved in the interpretation of laboratory tests that create a virtual mountain of paperwork. There is a great need for professionals with expertise in putting technology to its best use in patient care and research.

Another area of increasing interest involves the interaction of clinical pathology and the law. This is primarily related to the legal implications of expanding diagnostics (especially genetic testing). To qualify for this type of work, a pathologist will need law-related courses and possibly a degree in law.

The private corporate sector is also in need of professionals with both managerial and medical skills. Jobs are typically managerial positions found in newly started biotechnology companies, though they also can be found in larger pharmaceutical firms and businesses involved in diagnostic device research and development.

Pathologists advance by improving their skills and becoming experts in their field. In the academic world, they can advance to become full professors in colleges or universities, directors of research, or administrators, In the medical field, pathologists can advance to management positions in government agencies, private companies, or medical centers. For example, a highly experienced pathologist might advance to become the head of the pathology department in a large hospital. Another way to advance is to start an independent diagnostic laboratory, or become a consultant to private industry.

GETTING STARTED

THE BEST PLACE TO START FINDING A JOB in pathology is the job placement center at your university or medical school. Be sure to visit the center often. Recruiters will contact the placement center when they are coming to visit, and your school will post new job opportunity listings as they come up.

The next best source of information on potential job opportunities are your professors. Pathology professors are often practicing themselves or are actively involved in professional organizations where they have many contacts that may be helpful. Develop good relationships with your professors and ask that they let you know of any jobs that may be opening up.

Internships and work experience are an integral part of your education. In addition to obtaining vital hands-on experience in the field, it is common to use them as a stepping stone to future job positions. In these situations, you are making connections with people who have the power to hire you down the road. Make the most of these opportunities. Work hard, be enthusiastic about the work, and leave the best impression that you possibly can. Be sure to keep in touch with the people you work with so connections do not fade away.

Join regional and national pathology associations. The major pathology associations often have job boards and are good places for making job contacts. There are also many different organizations that are each devoted to a specific area of practice. Choose the ones that best match your future career plans. They may not have job boards, but they will have schedules for upcoming events on their websites. Attending pathology conferences is an excellent way to meet people in the field and make connections. It also looks great on your résumé. You can also find openings for pathologists listed in professional journals that are not published by associations.

You can apply directly to private firms, medical centers, colleges and universities, or government agencies that hire pathologists. Before you apply to any jobs, be sure that your résumé is polished and ready to go. Most colleges and universities offer career planning workshops, seminars, and one-on-one sessions with career counselors. Take advantage of these opportunities and sign up. You can ask your school's career guidance counselor and job placement center for help in preparing your résumé. You want it to highlight your strengths and to be presented in a professional format.

ASSOCIATIONS

■ College of American Pathologists
http://www.cap.org

■ American Pathology Foundation
https://www.apfconnect.org

■ American College of Veterinary Pathologists
http://www.acvp.org

■ American Phytopathological Society
http://www.apsnet.org

■ American Society for Clinical Pathology
www.ascp.org/content/Students

■ United States & Canadian Academy of Pathology
http://www.uscap.org/about

■ American Society of Cytopathology
http://www.cytopathology.org

PERIODICALS

■ The American Journal of Pathology
http://ajp.amjpathol.org

■ Modern Pathology
http://www.nature.com/modpathol/index.html

WEBSITES

■ Liaison Committee on Medical Education (LCME)
www.lcme.org

■ Intersociety Committee on Pathology Information (ICPI)
http://www.pathologytraining.org